Body Mutiny:
Surviving Nine Months of Extreme Morning Sickness

Jenna C. Schmitt

Library of Congress Cataloging-in-Publication Data

Schmitt, Jenna C.
  Body mutiny: surviving nine months of extreme morning sickness/Jenna C. Schmitt
      p. cm.
ISBN-13: 978-0-9774306-1-1 (pbk.: alk. paper)
ISBN-10: 0-9774306-1-8 (pbk.: alk. paper)
1. Morning sickness. 2. Schmitt, Jenna C. I. Title.

RG579.S36 2006
618.20092--dc22

                                    2006022786

Cover Design by Kelly Isola
Published by Acacia Publishing, Inc.
Phoenix, Arizona
www.acaciapublishing.com
Printed and Bound in the USA

Body Mutiny:
Surviving Nine Months of Extreme Morning Sickness

Jenna C. Schmitt

Edited by Monica Reeves VanDerWeide

Foreword by Julie Kwatra, M.D.

2006
Acacia Publishing, Inc.
Phoenix, Arizona

This book is solely dedicated to the mystery of pregnancy. This was my first and last pregnancy. It was full of suffering and agony, but I learned three profound things:

1) I love my Lord and my God, first and foremost

2) I love my husband more than ever

3) I discovered that doctors can be logical and compassionate (thanks, Dr. Kwatra)

The challenge now is to live my devotion.

God bless all you pregnant mothers, your families, and caregivers!

Foreword

Hyperemesis gravidarum. Even the name sounds ominous. These Greek and Latin words meaning "excessive nausea and vomiting of pregnancy" do not describe the usual morning sickness. Although a miserable experience for many, morning sickness is relatively harmless and often resolves three or four months into pregnancy. Hyperemesis gravidarum is a term reserved for the most severe cases of nausea and vomiting. It is so severe that the patient cannot eat. It is so severe that it can lead to dehydration, electrolyte imbalance, weight loss, and malnutrition. It often persists throughout the entire pregnancy, as it did in Jenna's case. It seems fitting that the word "gravidarum" (referring to pregnancy) comes from the Latin word gravis, meaning heavy or serious. This is truly a serious condition of pregnancy, and a heavy burden for those who suffer from it.

In earlier years, the mother's psychological state was felt to be the cause of this illness. We now know it is a physical disease, but the cause is not known. There is no cure. We can only treat the symptoms and side effects: drugs for nausea, IV fluids, and IV nutrition. Despite the best of medicine and the best intentions, this illness exacts a terrible toll from those afflicted with it. Fortunately, it is rare.

This book chronicles one woman's journey through the living hell of hyperemesis gravidarum. Jenna had one of the most extreme cases I have seen during my career as a physician. The theme of this book is not her physical and psychological torment, although both are understandable. Instead, what emerges from Jenna's prose is the miraculous endurance of the human spirit that can overcome every hardship.

We all celebrated Jenna's successful pregnancy outcome: a beautiful boy named Jay. As his life blooms, I hope the hyperemesis fades away into distant memory.

Julie Kwatra, MD

"Fare forward, travellers! Not escaping from the past
Into different lives, or into any future;
You are not the same people who left that station
Or who will arrive at any terminus,
While the narrowing rails slide together behind you;
And on the deck of the drumming liner
Watching the furrow that widens behind you,
You shall not think 'the past is finished'
Or 'the future is before us'."

*T.S. Eliot, from Four Quartets, "The Dry Salvages"

*Eliot, T.S. Four Quartets. T.S. Eliot Collected Poems 1909-1962. New York: Harcourt Brace & Company, 1963.

The Nature of Hyperemesis Gravidarum: Jenna's Story

According to most respected medical works, hyper-emesis gravidarum, or severe nausea and vomiting in pregnancy, is a rare condition, afflicting roughly one to two percent of all expectant mothers. It is characterized by "excessive" vomiting (more than five times daily), inability to ingest food and liquid, presence of key tones in urine (indication of starvation), and general gastric distress. Although I am no medical expert, I will share with you my experience and the resulting treatments.

I started to show signs of this wretched disorder at about four weeks of pregnancy and ended up in the emergency room after vomiting continuously for several days and becoming faint and dehydrated. I was given an IV antidote, which stopped the vomiting immediately, and was sent home with a prescription for Compazine pills. The pills did not work and I returned again to the emergency room a week later. Again the IV antidote, Anzamet, stopped the vomiting and I was sent home with a prescription for Tigan, after receiving a Tigan suppository in the hospital. Finally, my obstetrician became concerned, as I was unable to keep any food down and very little liquid. She had me try oral Zofran tablets as a last resort to hospitalization. These worked for about a week, and then I was sent to the maternity floor with severe dehydration.

I was admitted to the hospital at approximately seven weeks gestation. I tried more IV Anzamet, Tigan, Phenergan, Reglan, and was finally administered IV Zofran after each previous medication failed to stop the vomiting. The Reglan in particular caused terrible side effects, including a seizure-like reaction of involuntary muscle movement and hysteria. The IV Zofran seemed to keep the vomiting episodes down to less than ten per day and usually less than five. However, I tried to eat dry carbohydrates and could not keep any food and very little liquid down. The result was a continuous saline drip to keep me somewhat hydrated. Finally, after a two-week stay, my doctor became afraid of malnutrition and installed a central catheter (PICC line) into my arm, through which I could receive constant IV hydration and Zofran. She also ordered a regimen of TPN (total perinatal nutrition) to start through home nursing. During this time, my husband and I struggled not to terminate the pregnancy, and we decided to give the home health care a chance.

We maintained this schedule of IV Zofran, IV hydration, and TPN nutrition as I could not eat any solid food and could only drink small amounts of apple juice. Unfortunately, the vomiting cycle increased unbearably to more than 20 times a day. I was once again admitted to the hospital around the start of the second trimester. This visit resulted in my sedation by Ativan and use of Ambien and Paxil to help me sleep and gain strength.

Again we struggled with the termination issue and discovered we had until 22 weeks in the state of Arizona to make that decision final. My doctor also tried a steroid trial to control the severe nausea, which did not work. At this time, it was discovered that I had a damaged gallbladder, which would need to be removed immediately after birth or earlier if I developed an infection. Both the general surgeon and my obstetrician were unsure if the gallbladder problem contributed to the severity of the hyperemesis. I was discharged after a week's stay with some ease in the vomiting cycle.

Continuing on the IV schedule of home nursing, Zofran, and TPN, I began to suffer from severe heartburn and to vomit up large amounts of dried blood from a suspected tear in my esophagus. My obstetrician consulted with a gastric specialist, and I was placed on large amounts of Pepcid and Zantac via IV TPN. About halfway through my second trimester, I developed a very high fever (105 degrees), chills, and extreme muscle aches that sent me back to the hospital. My doctor suspected an infected gallbladder, but in fact I had developed a dangerous staph infection in my PICC line. I was treated with strong IV antibiotics in the hospital and at home after my fever subsided. At this point, my husband and I decided to continue with the pregnancy and put the termination issue behind us, despite my hyperemesis ordeal.

The TPN and IV Zofran treatment continued into my early third trimester. I began to eat very small amounts of food and took increasingly large doses of oral Zantac and Prilosec to control severe heartburn. I also tried accupuncture treatment to ease the hyperemesis, although it did not work. My vomiting remained under relative control (fewer than ten times daily) and I was able to reduce the amount of IV Zofran received daily. The PICC dressings caused me to develop several serious skin infections and lesions, one of which was an E Coli infestation on my left arm. Again I was treated with IV antibiotics, which worked well. After several placement problems with the PICC line and the increasing risk of infection, my obstetrician decided to pull the line entirely and see if I could eat on my own.

The PICC line was finally removed at week 32 of my pregnancy, along with the TPN nutrition. I still remained on the IV Zofran, although it was received through a needle in my skin rather than through a central line.

I also continued to take large oral doses of Zantac, Paxil, and Prilosec to advert an ulcer and to control nausea. The vomiting had decreased to every other day and the nausea seemed to be less severe, although constantly present. Midway through my eighth month of pregnancy, it was decided that I would carry until the 37th week and be induced to end my misery and avoid any further infections. The baby continued to thrive and gain significant weight through all of this and experienced no fetal complications.

I struggled mightily to keep food and sufficient nourishment down despite staying on the 24-hour Zofran pump at 36 weeks. At my next doctor's visit, I was again spilling key tones into my urine and having a difficult time even getting out of bed. The OB decided to perform an amniocentesis to see if the baby's lungs were ready. If so, I would stay in the hospital and be induced at 36 weeks and two days gestation. Unfortunately for us, the baby wasn't quite ready so we were sent home with an induction date of August 16th, at 37 weeks and two days gestation. At this point in the pregnancy, the baby would be considered full-term and ready to deliver. It was planned that Cytotek would be administered on the 16th to start the induction. My cervix was relatively thick, and I was only dilated to one centimeter.

My husband and I were called to the hospital's OB triage unit in the middle of the night on the 16th to begin induction. A cervical softening medicine was introduced at 2:30 a.m. and contractions began almost immediately. No real progress was made although the contractions became stronger and more insistent throughout the next day. I progressed to three centimeters by the early evening and Pitocin was commenced. Later that same evening, I requested an epidural that lasted effectively throughout the night and gave me the opportunity to sleep. By morning, however, my cervix was still thick and dilation had not progressed. Our OB broke my bag of waters to speed the process.

During the second full day of induced labor, the epidural began to wear off and several "top-offs" failed to produce the required pain relief.

Later in the afternoon, I began to feel feverish and strong attacks of vomiting and nausea ensued. The fever rose to 103 degrees and the baby's heartbeat rose dangerously along with it. It was determined that I had acquired a uterine infection. The persistent hyperemesis and the stress of such a strong and long labor produced more relentless attacks of vomiting. These problems compounded the situation and in the 47th hour of labor it was decided that a C-section would solve the problem. I had only progressed to six centimeters and my cervix was not thinned out sufficiently.

We quickly moved to the operating room, where my blood was typed and crossed in case a transfusion was needed. The epidural was once again topped off and worked well through the first part of surgery. Unfortunately, I began to feel sharp pains of cutting during the latter part of the operation. I was given massive doses of narcotics to dull the pain, which quelled my anxiety but did not relieve the sensations. The baby was taken out and a tubal ligation was performed. After leaving the OR, I continued to experience very painful contractions brought on by the high levels of Pitocin still in my body. Morphine failed to ease the misery and I was given IV Ativan, which knocked me out and brought on much needed rest.

I healed from the C-section very quickly and remained in the hospital for the rest of the week on IV antibiotics. The baby had to stay in the NICU due to an infection and water in the lungs (a common complication of C-section surgery). The nausea had miraculously disappeared by the morning after surgery. I returned home and continued to take my large doses of Zantac and Prilosec to control the lingering hyperemesis-related heartburn. Alternate bouts of constipation and loose bowels marked my entrance into the world of eating again. We welcomed a healthy but tired baby home after one week and two days in the NICU.

Almost 2 ½ weeks after the delivery, my appetite came back with a vengeance, and I regained my taste buds that had been dulled by past vomiting. I still relied on medication to control heartburn after meals and had trouble digesting meats and vegetables. My faithful OB referred me to a gastric specialist to address the possible esophageal tear. The endoscopy showed several microscopic tears which would heal on their own. I discontinued the anti-acid and heartburn medications about a month after delivery.

Finally, my fatigue disappeared and I was able to talk short walks around our neighborhood and start household chores again like cooking and laundry (too bad!). It was an incredible relief to begin to forget the days and nights of interminable nausea, vomiting, and excessive salivation. I was able to complete this book without physically relieving the hyperemesis symptoms during the writing process. Life as a non-pregnant woman was much sweeter than I had remembered it.

***For more information on hyperemesis gravidarum and support for those who suffer from it, please consult a respected hyperemesis website, www.hyperemesis.org or contact the author at jenna@extrememorningsickness.com

Week One

My mother thinks that the term "knocked up" is coarse,
vulgar, and gross.
It doesn't apply to marital conception,
just premarital action.

There's a gaping irony between a thing so feared by one
but so desired by two.
Being a person of extremes,
I see it as a natural turn of events:
a moment of infinite possibility,
which has never been experienced
except maybe in our earliest forms.

What have we forgotten that we originally knew?

The laughter
and the rain showers
and the dust settle so quickly
on the pages
of childhood, grown
wary by experience into adulthood,
expecting results and fruition by our own hand
and not hearing the music,
which has always and will ever more
play in our stupid, senseless heads

In the green corner bedroom,
which was chilly in the winter
and stifling in the summer,
the sunny curtains were sometimes
covered with frost
driven by perpendicular winds

There was a lamp with a carousel
pulled by ponies and kittens---
I wasn't supposed to wind it, but I did
and wound it unbearably tight one afternoon,
so tight I could hear the protesting chinks
from virgin springs

It played a meaningless song off key
at a good pace for an hour,
and then it seemed to run out and lost my attention.
I left the room for play and returned to sleep, falling
into an innocent sleep, imagining what would become
and forgetting what was, when---
A SINGLE NOTE sounded in my head
and I jumped up,
startled and relieved
that it was just the song
that I had started

For years in the green room, that carousel sang,
even though the music was no longer heard;
now it probably lies in a backyard junk pile
under books with broken bindings
and cracked glasses:
ALL
are touched lovingly by the Hand
that continues the song
in its imperfection,
not playing for anyone
but heard

Week Two

The black appointment book has many small squares
with countless scribblings, lists, and revisions:
notes are crossed out and re-written,
dotted with red and black ink.
All of my weekly goals
and warnings are intermixed
and practically illegible in this book,
at the start of December...

A sharp little bird
with quickly beating wings
draws us into the nest
through our volition
and feeds us with the passion
of her own experience

She regurgitates book wisdom
and common sense
into our open, unknowing mouths,
and we are content to be fed
and confident in our purpose.
Content and confident too
are those who surround us,
far ahead on their paths
and happy to show off
swollen accomplishments

while the rest of us sit
with flat bellies,
HUNGRY
for what lies
ahead.

The figuring, the guessing, and the monitoring
take center stage in ten days,
and the act becomes
calculated and prepossessed,
even though the likewise is said.

Despite the
FOOLISHNESS
and
PRESUMPTUOUSNESS
and
ARROGANCE
of
me. . .

Love comes to us
and winds its whispery fingers
around the longing,
silencing the prayers for completion
and prompting the ticking by of hours
until I start to pay attention
to what is outside
of pure desire.

Week Three

The day I took my first riding lesson
was a humbling one.
I thought I would just jump on
and gallop off:
EFFORTLESSLY,
POETICALLY,
a natural talent to be sure

But I had failed to realize
that this fantasy required something
I had never possessed,
and that was:
BALANCE

The day I took my first riding lesson,
I lost the reins
(well, I was denied them)
and the horse went round and round,
attached to a person who praised the horse
but who screamed at my lack
of coordination

Fighting against
involuntary movement and gravity,
I struggled without reins:

pitching off the back of the hindquarters;
rolling off the side;
bouncing up the shoulders;
falling off the neck;
Luckily, the horse was kind enough
to step around me
and move on.

One magic day I discovered the mystery of the trot,
and the jarring and jangling went away.
I felt as proud and regal as a queen in a parade,
my mount prancing as if on air
and I glided majestically with him
for one spectacular moment. . .
until everything broke
and I flopped off of the side
AGAIN.

But the moments of magic grew longer;
I learned to halt my expectations
and just FEEL---
there was no more suspicion
of my own inadequacy
or of the horse's perceived ill will,
and lo, and behold,
I took the reins.

That was no
cheap ticket to freedom.

I was warned that
what was so given
could also be taken away.

Those reins were delicate threads
that would break if I pulled too hard
or leaned on them for support,
and the horse always had the final say

This is how I learned to ride
and to fall
and to ride again

Week Four

Into the hazy sunshine
of an Arizona winter,
sleep shortens long afternoons;
I welcome these unexpected naps
but I also puzzle over them.
Gentle slumber falls over me
like a warm blanket,
during far warmer mid days

Lunar cycles point to change
and the inner cycle responds,
sending out telegraphs of pain
and notable discomfort.

I tolerate all of this
as the normal monthly occurrence
of corrupt hormones
UNTIL
expectation slowly leaks through
a guise of nonchalance and skepticism
that I normally hold near.

A spontaneous moment of discovery:
quick tears and then disbelief;
John and I check and recheck the results
until our budget is much challenged

We feel, on the surface, wild exhilaration,
but our true happiness originates from
a much deeper source.

Two parallel lines
will run on forever if
they are left unchecked---
and so will the human thought,
roaming and rediscovering itself,
born into the origin of things.

The Divine touches our dreaming thoughts,
weaving the same whispery web of love
that we have known before
into more intricate
and unbelievable designs.

Week Five

Two towheads and happy neighbors
arrive for a winter dinner.
We hide our celebratory intent,
content only to become acquainted with them---
Among holiday lights and merry houses,
we feast together.

I nose down to the village display
and see that snow flies,
and that holiday parties gather.
Over all of it, a lone dog
near the dark castle
stands peaceful sentry.

A familiar aura settles
as we dine sumptuously;
the roast simmers
and wine falls roundly
into goblets.
It seems almost a medieval affair,
alit with carnal warmth and filling bellies,
peppered with tales of music lessons
and the more humorous demands
of virtuous dating.

We are all the wiser
for our homespun creation;
John and I are pleased with the aura,
snug in the goal achieved,
and excited by the intimacy
that fans our flame.

These guests,
these mystery neighbors,
become an innermost part
of our lives this evening,
evolving into friends
and applauding our announcement.

Every eye shines with joy and wonder.

We retire to the candlelit living room,
enticed by creamy and dreamy chocolates,
carefully plucking our favorites with fingertips.
Drawn from couches and chairs onto the floor,
we join in a sort of familiar union---
the towheads,
happy neighbors,
and we two,
fall into separate visions
of what will be.

Week Six

Things submerged beneath waters,
especially deep ocean waters,
have a devious way
of making themselves known.

They do not
SURPRISE
or
DELIGHT
or
THRILL
or
YIELD
to us

They
FRIGHTEN
and
DISORIENT
and
LURK
and
SICKEN
and run cold fear
from their depths
to our own.

These are things of experience,
startlingly discovered
by human impetuousness
in moments of carefree play

FREEDOM breaks,
and we learn that
we must always take care,
especially in deep water.

I journey backward in my mind's eye
to Leeside Beach,
a place of prelapsarian wonder
I once knew---
it was a typical Massachusetts beach
lacking a sandy bottom,
but it was blessed with smooth stones,
lack of seaweed at high tide,
and bath-like water temperature
(thanks to the good folks
at New England Power
across the way)

Our aunts and uncles and older cousins
swam in the night out to the wooden raft;
there they reclined and surveyed winking lights
on the Mount Hope Bay Bridge,
and the spectacle of Fall River
laid out along the hillside.

Nothing disturbed but the hum
of the soft brackish tide.

I would dream of Leeside
while I was in Michigan,
trapped in Midwestern snowy winters
and saltless lakes.

My dreams were always full of
oceanic perfection.

One summer at Leeside,
early in the summer
(that's always the time),
a morning backstroke
shattered it all.

Something deathly soft and encircling
stung like a wasp
in between my shoulders. . .

I bounded to the beach in one step,
burning on the outside
and wounded on the inside.
But I never saw the offender
and spent the remainder
of that day
on hot and itchy sands.

Week Six, Part Two

Hardly a day had passed
when my childish short memory
relinquished the thought---
It did not flutter away like a cinder;
it dropped like a brick.

Again the tides brought me from the shore,
this time perched on top of the water
and on top of an inflatable raft:
my eyes skimmed methodically
from leeward to sand

There was a complete absence of innocence---
I had already been tainted
AND
up from the bottom they arose:

PURPLISH BATTALIONS

TENS IN NUMBER

PULSATING LIKE NAKED ORGANS

INSIDE OUT

SOFTER THAN WATER

GAPING RINGS AND ORIFICES

Frilly appendages fingered up the sides
of my raft.

They rose beyond the imagination
and through the flat realm of experience
that had always made
me its master.

The merciful tide pushed me to shore
and when my eyes were fully open,
there was a three-dimensional world.

Vision, true vision,
PIERCED
and became reality
at Leeside beach.

I saw the rusty bent pipe
protruding from eel grass;

I saw a half-sunken rowboat
crawling with hundreds
of multi-legged crabs;

I saw tide pools swirling glumly
with cloudy residue;

I saw more than the occasional tampon
floating limply in tepid water,
half submerged from view

I saw creatures oozing in such pools
that were almost too deviant
to remember...

I saw ghostly carcasses
with too many heads and too few joints,
their dried intestines crumbling into the murk;

I saw tubular round worms with
waving fingers and sucking mouths;

I saw an unidentified mollusk
with its guts splayed wide open,
shredded by skittery sea spiders...

My stomach turned,
and I backed away into
the shadows of seaside trees,
the beach becoming smaller and smaller
in my new line of vision.

Week Six, Part Three

In time, I sought larger vessels
to transport me across many seas.
Our sailboat rose high above
the surface of churning waves,
detached from beneath.

To think I was well protected
became my defense,
all the while clashing
with the irony that
I was not.

With the blinders strung tightly,
I could hear silent horrors
passing beneath the keel:
spiky sea-mines disengaged
from an unknown bottom
and bumped menacingly
against the hull;

Giant propellers from
uncharted wreckages
pierced the sky
and threatened
our buoyancy;

I saw man-made and stilt-legged structures,
oil rigs and landing platforms
rising up out of the fog,
their legs bracing against
unsteady reefs;

They towered hundreds of feet above the mist,
their sheer hulk threatening
to demolish us all.

Week Seven

The significant year of 2004
rolls across my consciousness again,
shaking the grip of memory.

Moments retrace
across a bottomless bowl
of soup steaming before me,
smooth and glistening on top,
hiding its golden ingredients
from view.

I think again of these things
as I eat New Year's leftovers:
SUDDENLY
the stomach turns deeply
and the eyes turn inward

I realize that I chew
the fatty sinews of an animal
that was last week's feast

AND

I inhale at the recognition
of the onset of the unknown,
rising. . .

The thing that was submerged imperceptibly
now moves to the surface
and hangs on.

Week Seven, Part Two

Morning light filters off-yellow
through our bedroom shades;
it is a flat color without spark,
the reassuring depths of
Phoenix sunlight.

Forced by sheer need to use the bathroom,
I slip from our bed into the solitary room
that houses the throne.

My gaze swings the cubicle and the dull carpet:
there seem to be welcome puffs
of air conditioning blasting down from above,
cool in contrast to my sticky brow

When I turn my head, things shift like vertigo---
and my belly
FLOPS
down off an unseen edge;
drool releases,
followed by a full-body heave
which elevates me well off of the throne.

Into the depths of a white wastebasket
I retch boundlessly and enthusiastically without yield---

In fact, I retch joyfully with every muscle,
strained from shoulder to toe,
all in obeisance to the great and holy
demands of early life.

My head swirls and
I feel as if I am an honored vessel
of divine consecration,
glowing like the Madonna
in my lavatory splendor

I resolve to be humble and accepting,
happy to bear discomfort and
eager to bend the obstinate ego
to a higher love:
"Not my will but thine"

I glisten regally at the very thought of it.

These glorious moments of sacred contortion
soon fill my days with the same results:
BULGING EYES
RAGGED BREATHS
and
CELLULAR STRAINING

Prolonged retching within the bowels of self
soon voids up any arrogance that remains.

Within the depths
of a half-conscious dream,
I hear words in my ear
that I do not understand.

Compassion has come to bear me up,
as the darkness of knowing
starts to descend.

Week Eight

Listening to a school band
is like witnessing a traffic accident
in slow motion.

Melody and harmony are horribly mum
beneath a cacophonous racket of:
SHRILLING FLUTES
SQUAWKING CLARINETS
BLATTING SAXES
WHINY STRINGS
SHOUTING BRASS
BELCHING TUBAS
FARTING HORNS
and at the conclusion,
the ill-timed thump of the bass drum,
miserably measures behind
the whole crowd.

At this point, the conductor hides his face
and sweats buckets of shame,
but tone-deaf parents just revel
in the sheer mastery
of it all.

There is an addictive chaos
to this sort of musicianship.

The sheer noise ceases time
and strangles attention from even
the most resistant listeners.

Some year or two later,
when maturity sets in,
the budding young instrumentalists
learn the rigors of tuning and proper pitch.

It starts as an artificial process,
with a lone semi-competent flutist
or string player adjusting a B flat
to an electronic tuning machine;
if the gauge reads steady, the pitch is pure.

Any wobbling produces a nauseating clash of tones.

Once practice grants this musician
the ability to hit the pitch
(to whack it out of the park),
it is a moment of pure simplicity
imitated by the band in full chord.

The conductor cues forth the song and
in a drop of serenity and pure power,
the chord chimes out full and right,
flowing from the top to the bottom

Hearts stir in unison as an orchestra is born.

Week Nine

Harmony in the midst of chaos
takes on a whole new meaning
when it's trapped within the human body.

We return again to my proud maternal discomfort,
and find it rapidly descending into utter misery...

The body usually keeps us contained:
it arranges the jumble of intestines,
sets the tempo of its own electrical system,
and generally acts as a marvelous thermostat

But this body, my body, carries a passenger
that leaves no room to spare for me.

The point of entry becomes a wacky revolving door
of rapid entry and furious exit.

I puke in our bushes;

I spray random trees and cacti;

I become a menace at the Barnes & Noble Bookstore,
permanently destroying their carpet and
defacing their entryway;

I become a motor vehicular threat:
left hand drive, mouth vomit
into right hand bag;

I dirty Scottsdale's finest parks and walkways;

I gag and flee grocery stores, desperately trying
to hold myself in;

I christen
PARKED VEHICLES
BREATHING CREATURES
HOUSEHOLD APPLIANCES
A VARIETY OF FABRICS
HOLY PLACES
and
MUNDANE SPACES

The equal opportunity vomiting
sends me to the emergency room
and results in a preliminary diagnosis of:
NAUSEA AND VOMITING IN PREGNANCY (NVP)

During this vital decision-making process,
I limp around the waiting room
with my Tupperware barf-bucket
(alas, so many Tupperware
have fallen since then),
glaring at the charge nurse
for nearly four hours

My husband corrals my pacing
and simmers with rage at the
SLOW
SLOW
grindings of the medical cog

Finally I am placed on a stretcher
and receive kind but conflicting advice:
"crackers by the bedside, but no carbohydrates;
sodas good, but no carbonation;
sugary sweets encouraged, but no fruit juice permitted..."

The ER doc shrugs at these riddles
and sets me up with an IV Anzamet drip,
some Ativan for mental health,
and good old-fashioned sedatives.

SUDDENLY
the light inside blinks on and darkness ascends:
instant relief is full of the
grace of the Holy Spirit.

I am again a proud martyr for the act of conception.

Floaty giggles arise from the throat,
while my warm and delicious arms reach for John;
I beg for some sweet lovemaking
right there on the spot...

And my heart sings forth again, full of motherly song.

Week Ten

Well, folks, when the show's over
the curtain is sure to fall,
shrouding the stage
in darkness once again.

Such is my brief relief from the cantankerous self;
the Compazine prescribed has the power of a damp Kleenex,
shredded into trillions by a gale force blast.

The little bird is not pleased at my appearance---
she flutters over my sallow face and lost poundage;
she fusses over my non-existent blood pressure;
she clucks at my newly acquired Tupperware barf-bucket

HANDFULS OF ZOFRAN SAMPLES
(pricey little meds used
to soothe vomiting chemo patients),
MEDICAL FACT
(the fetus takes what it needs),
and
POSITIVE STATISTICS
(relief by twelve weeks)
placate John and me.

The cranky vomiting acquires
a new and prettier name at this point:
HYPEREMESIS GRAVIDARUM
(severe nausea and vomiting in pregnancy)

We feel important to have such
a noble Latinate diagnosis!

John and I fly out of the obstetrical nest,
chiding the stork but thanking
our little wise sparrow...

Week Eleven

Ritual is a strange master---
when our human will is incapacitated,
we become senseless robots and
genuflect like mannequins,
thoughtlessly crossing ourselves:
We even dare to consume salvation
like it is a fast food meal!

Action
DEVOID OF THOUGHT
DIVORCED FROM SPIRIT
RENT FROM DESIRE
is just poisonous repetition.

The cruelty of life
often expedites this separation,
stealing the warmth from our flesh
and narrowing our vision to a pinpoint.

I stumble in semi-darkness, numbly perpetuating
actions that are driven only
by animal hunger and thirst

EAT
VOMIT
DRINK

VOMIT
SLEEP
VOMIT
NAUSEA
NAUSEA
VOMIT

My body stinks in its own decay,
and the very protein in my cells
spills out. . .

We used to argue in lofty tones
about five-paragraph form in graduate school:
my favorite wiry-haired professor said
that without this form,
an essay was merely a puddle

Most of us held fast to this position,
but not because we were intimidated
by her intellect:
We were trained in this form,
and saw the unity and coherence
it produced. . .

Now my body is merely a puddle, a dysfunctional muddle.

The little bird swoops down
and places me in a large white house.
It is a place full of friendly angels
who poke at withered veins

and ease a slim blue catheter
into my beating heart.

The swell of a nauseated ocean
makes me dumb and hysterical;
I writhe in a tiny little hole of self-loathing
while the little invader sleeps within my depths,
THRIVING
while I starve
from the inside out.

Week Twelve

For two weeks I stay in the big white house:
John is my constant companion,
and Gerry from our church comes by
to talk sense into my senseless head.

My contempt grows for the invisible being,
(now the size of a grain of rice)
deep within my pelvis;
it triggers a flood of rising hormones
which speak evil lies to my brain,
bringing on the ceaseless vomiting.

I watch no T.V.,
read no books,
and make very little conversation.
I only stare at the big-numbered clock,
counting
SECONDS
MINUTES
HOURS
DAYS
and I pray for the death of something
that triggers the whole cycle
of inner madness.

Termination would be the end of it all,
a release from the deadly trap
that has been sprung

I might enter into its unknown and disbelieved territory,
a thought shunned before it is realized.

The drugs drip endlessly,
and late at night I hear a nameless voice
telling me that I can go now if I must---
but the sadness of not being here
would ache in the empty faces of the people
that I would leave behind,
and in that of the beloved man
who has created life with me.

Instead I choose to wait
and watch the clock tick on
at two in the morning,
in the new year of 2004. . .

It is also the new year of a life
that is only a yolk,
but our genes and love
flourish within it

The love of self pulls painfully away,
as scabs off of fresh wounds
of the heart.

Week Thirteen

At the end of our stay in the big white house,
food is my sworn enemy---
I try toasted white bread
but choke when it comes up
in big wet clumps, making me gag

I am wracked with hunger pains
but appetite sickens me more.

The little bird gives up
and she decides that my meals
(and the fetus's meals)
will consist of only intravenous nutrition---
it's the perfect diet when so many mothers
chose imperfect pregnancy diets:
CHEESEBURGERS WITH EXTRA CHEESE
and
GALLONS OF ROCKY ROAD
and
PINTS OF GREASY CHINESE NOODLES---
but there will be none
of that food for me.

Instead, this synthetic nourishment
drips into my body;
once it starts, the hunger fades away

and it's just as if I had never eaten
in the first place.

That normal part of life departs,
and I linger on in the darkness of our bedroom,
sleeping through the days and praying for early nights

John makes an extraordinary metamorphosis
from accountant by day to nurse by evening;
he fights constantly to calibrate the pumps
and to maintain the scheduled dosing
that regulates my maternity.

Then there are the idiocies
of home health management:
late night deliveries
AND
incorrect supplies
AND
unanswered phone messages
AND
wailing alarms
AND
incompetent nurse visits.

The tension mounts as we suffer through
days beyond the first trimester.

Week Fourteen

The childhood vault of memory
is a place I occupy for a majority
of my conscious days;
I reject the present because
I just can't deal with it...

However, I CAN check in when I need to,
like when the natural urge to expel waste arises,
or when John needs cooperation,
or when the nurse arrives to evaluate me...

But usually, I just muse in semi-consciousness
through the endless daylight hours,
and I recall the horseback rides
and college parties
and moments of freedom
I used to enjoy.

Unconsciousness offers no creative outlet for me:
I sleep I but never dream,
since my dreams are all played out
during the day.

Each weekday passes without a thought
of its passing; unfortunately,
the weekends sting harder because John is home,

and I am constantly reminded of my poor state
by his 24-hour care

I perform the fine art of vomiting
with excruciating frequency:

I CAN'T BREATHE
I CAN'T BREATHE
I CAN'T BREATHE

But I don't panic;
I just do what is necessary
and bring up more bodily fluids,
all while trying to recall
pleasanter moments
from the past.

Week Fifteen

It's amusing that in times such as this,
in the grips of this hyperemesis disease,
my mind travels back
to the one activity
I hated the most while growing up:
SAILING.

It was a forced march on weekends
when my father and his "crew"
(my mother and me)
would sail a small lake all afternoon,
FROM TOP TO BOTTOM
FROM BOTTOM TO TOP
passing the same landmarks
and seeing the same watery undulations
every weekend.

I prayed to the god of rain each Saturday;
I begged for a respite while staying
Friday night at my friend's house.
In the early morning, I would run to the window,
scanning for raindrops and hoping
for the miraculous funnel cloud
or toxic gas spill
or tri-state traffic disaster...

Unfortunately,
I was seldom spared from the Saturday ritual,
and weekly I witnessed my father
fight the unremarkable seas
of Lake Wawasee in Northern Indiana;
perhaps he was imagining Cape Cod's waters
or his nautical trek to Bermuda...

Back when we lived in Massachusetts,
I don't remember sailing as a dreaded burden:
instead, it seemed almost a mythical adventure,
with romantic ports on the Vineyard,
and indigenous gifts acquired along the way.

This was all part of the adventure
of traversing the great body of water
known as the Atlantic Ocean.

Week Sixteen

The marvelous adventure of sailing the open ocean
caught my imagination in its web,
when we lived on the East Coast---
my father drove the boat hard against off-shore winds,
and my mother jumped to adjust the sails. . .

Being pretty young, I often stayed down below,
propping myself against the heeled-over hull
as I worked steadily on coloring books,
spreading Crayola vibrancy on the pages.

Periodically I would emerge
on the slippery deck, which was draped with sail lines
(in nautical terms called "sheets"),
and littered with winch handles and empty soda cans

Discarded tuna sandwiches and
snack-size bags of chips lay on the deck;
consequently, every surface burgeoned
with black flies, after our many hours
spent out on the water.

In brisk wind, the boat sliced smoothly
through the waves as we meandered
the New England coastline,
cutting across Buzzard's Bay
into the open Atlantic.

In bad wind or dead calm, the boat bobbled clumsily
as we puttered into the bay and dodged motorized crafts,
hoping for a breeze to break the monotony
of glassy seas and kelp flotillas

MYSTERIOUSLY
and often in the midst of a dead calm,
a thick and soupy fog would descend on us,
fouling up my father's navigations
and making my mother nervous.

But the sight of this mist filled me with wonderment
at what encircled our boat.

The vestiges of land were gone
and a personal puddle of water surrounded us.
The greater realm of the sea lay outside of our eyes,
with its natural and man-made obstacles,
waiting to surprise us and maybe trip us up.

Usually these objects were fairly harmless,
like beer bottles or floating driftwood:
as the fog would become denser,
my father would send my mother out to the far bow
for her to crouch with a compact air-horn,
trying to warn massive freighters
and speeding pleasure boats alike
of our existence.

It was an exciting time, waiting to see
what would emerge from the fog:
usually it was nothing but gradually revealed
forms of land or nearby boats,
both signaling our release from fog soup.

However, from time to time,
a dark ship bulkhead would steam past rapidly,
uncomfortably close to the sailboat's hull,
and rock our whole vessel in its wake---

I was amazed
that it could appear instantly
out of what I saw as nothing.

Week Seventeen

Through the days and nights of darkness,
and in the perceived darkness of my own mind,
I live only in memory
while the real world slides past.

Outsiders who call me cannot even begin to understand
this hyperemesis misery.

I do not hold this against them,
but it alienates me nonetheless:
every breath I draw is preoccupied with vomit,
and my veins are filled with artificial nourishment

One Sunday afternoon,
I sit in bed with my husband and I can't stand it any longer---
I need a mental break,
A RESPITE
AN OASIS
from the parched desert of dehydration hell
that chokes. . .

I want to yank the line out of my vein
and sever the very tie that keeps me alive,
making me a prisoner to the incubation march

In teary hysteria,
I phone the on-call doctor and once again,
we enter the white house
in search of some solace.

Week Eighteen

It's astounding what the mind will conjure up
when it's warped and disrupted,
like a train derailed from the tracks...

T.S. Eliot says that we are never the same persons
who leave the train station:
time passes so quickly behind us
that we can forget who we were
and get hopelessly swallowed up
in the present.

In the friendly white house again,
I am under the merciful influence of Ativan,
which crosses my eyes and sends
nonsense words tumbling
from my lips

This medicated unreality soothes me
and I sleep, exhausted from the effort of vomiting
and temporarily relieved from a tormented existence...

But I DO exist!

And I am finally free from the responsibility
of putting on a brave face,
of pretending that it is better than it truly is---

I can no longer speak lies that are kinder
for others to hear than the sharp truth of the moment.

Vulnerability to other people's opinions
makes me realize how delicate I truly am.

And I can cry freely
for the first time in months
because I KNOW my own suffering.

The outsiders suddenly file in:

THE TRIM DIETICIAN
THE HOPEFUL PHYSICIAN
THE EAGER SURGEON
THE EFFICIENT NURSE
THE DISTURBED VISITOR

All of these gradually meander into
the big room in which I stay,
surrounded by mothers
with real flesh-and-blood babies.

I have to remind myself that
these others are the PLAYERS on my team,
NOT the opponents: so I fall into their care
without a peep of dissention, and I tolerate
their last-ditch efforts to bring me SOME comfort.

*There is strain in the voice of the phone caller
and in the face of the family member,
when both realize that it's so much worse
than they could have imagined.*

*Others remain outside this tight circle
of what I term "hyperemesis hell":
even the little bird is no closer to me
than the history of her last patient*

*I AM ALONE
to fight the monster that doesn't
play by the rulebook and takes the cheapest shots
when I am at my weakest...*

Week Nineteen

This stay in the big white house
stretches beyond days into weeks,
without any real improvement
in my condition. . .

My attitude, however, has changed:
I begin to feel the passage of time
and note that the clock's hands DO move

Pregnancy is not a permanent state;
the body's evolving form shakes me
from the depths of self-pity into the grit of resolve,
as I vow to search for goodness
in the middle of my suffering.

I now watch the T.V.
and I view the news half-heartedly;
I also put in random threads on my latch-hook project,
trying to recreate the playful Labrador
that romps on the cover of the box.

My nausea and my intent
to distract myself from it
shift advantage like players in a chess match
BUT
repetitious activity begins to lift the mental fog

We prepare to go home to our ready-made hospital,
which is full of I.V. poles and a fridge burgeoning with:

INTRAVENOUS FOOD MIXTURES
SALINE FLUSHES
VITAMIN ADDITIVES
ZOFRAN SYRINGES
PUMP TUBING

Now, I live only for the passage of time
and the mercy
of an inevitable birth.

Week Twenty

Our house smells stale from the stench of misery;
it is no longer a "normal" place
that wafts fabric softener
and baking cookies
and toast,
all with an aura
of comfort mixed in. . .

I return home and remember the vomiting places
of the past weeks, resuming my rest
in our shaded bedroom
during the long days.

The medical supplies vastly overwhelm
the baby stuff: a lone fuzzy onesie hangs
from the old dresser in what has yet to become
THE BABY'S ROOM.

Our priest arrives and graces the house
with his jovial, massive form---
He blesses me with the anointed holy oil of healing,
and incense fills the upstairs hall,
brushing against each crucifix that guards the doorway
to each upstairs room

Before, I felt that the holy relics
and ancient prayers had failed me,
leaving me trapped inside a hopelessly wasted body:
BUT NOW, life deep inside defies the illness
and starts to STIR

This small hope prompts me to turn
from the lure of a loaded .45
into a state of waiting for grace to descend.

I will try to expect "delayed joy" at the end of the journey,
a kind of quiet jubilation that would have never been known
without the sorrow

Thus my realization of an end sustains what food cannot.

Week Twenty One

My mother arrives to greet us,
as we make yet another return from the white house:
she is poised and ready to assert
her motherly rights over our
chaotic quarters...

We gratefully encourage her to do so,
and she goes right to work:

SHE DOES AND FOLDS THE LAUNDRY;

SHE VACUUMS THE DOGS' CRATES;

SHE ORGANIZES OUR CLOSETS;

SHE PREPARES JOHN'S FAVORITE MEATLOAF;

I tease her that she is one happy domestic slave.

We aren't used to having a healthy woman around;
it is odd to live with someone who
takes showers on a daily basis,
and someone who can eat
without the aid of an I.V. bag.

I think she is shocked to be exposed to our misery firsthand.

She cringes when John shows her my daily medical routine,
afraid of poisoning me with the good medicine.
We try to assure her that it can't happen,
and that my body takes on that malicious role
all by itself. . .

It is not normal for a thirty-year-old woman to live
the life of an elderly infirm;
it is merely a status quo existence.

We live in constant fear of relapse
or infection, doing everything we can
to avoid a collapse
into complete despair.

Week Twenty Two

My mother's presence inspires us
to reach beyond our constricted lives
into the land of the living;
MIRACULOUSLY
something amazing occurs,
and I can step out into the strong sunlight,
leaving our dim house behind.

Mom and I venture out into the mountains,
to the other side of the Valley of the Sun,
into a city of fountains.
We wander down an entire avenue dedicated
to towers of rushing water, in all sorts
of ingenious and artistic positions.

I wish I could float in one of those pools
or immerse myself in a pond,
or just sit under the spray of the aquatic statues;
there's just no way to rid myself
of the stink of regurgitation

Even away from our sick house, I still see everything
rising to the surface, again and again. . .

I need a baptism from the deep sins
that my body commits;

I want to eat again and feel the old tingle
of flavor and of desire I used to enjoy;

I want to be an independent being
and sustain myself!

Feeling these desires anew,
I attempt to eat
as Mom and I sit under a shady tree
in the town of fountains.

I eat one Cheerio at a time,
and they drop like petrified dust
into my stomach, which has been virgin
for nearly the entire pregnancy

I wash these few O's down with weak lemonade,
the only hydration I can take past my lips. . .

Week Twenty Three

Time drags its feet,
crawling along and creeping without much purpose:
finally, it rolls my gestational calendar
to the start of the third trimester.

Easter comes and goes in a flash;
it's usually a spiritual holiday of welcome renewal,
but this time around, it's just another
unremarkable day to be tolerated,
just another trip out of the sick house.

We lunch in on Easter day with the family,
and I watch everyone ingesting his or her brunch food
without a conscious thought to the whole miraculous process;
to me, eating holds the mystique of ascending Mount Everest
without supplemental oxygen
or riding bareback across the Arabian Desert

For me, eating is a feat, not an instinctual activity.

I console myself with some cranberry juice
and a piece of ripe fruit or two;
I feel these things settle none too happily
into a highly medicated stomach,
vexing my already preoccupied thoughts

Body Mutiny

They just don't get it, these outsiders,
and even those people so close to us...

Are they in denial or just too busy to see what's going on?

They continue their dinners out at the Club;
they continue to live by the demands
of the practical and social calendar,
while John and I float aimlessly
in our own private Sargasso Sea

We find ourselves cast away
by these happy and distant faces,
and we are SO tired of being mired
in the seaweed of our own morose discontent.

Perhaps we intentionally distance ourselves
and set sail without anyone else's push:
or maybe that's the explanation
with which they comfort themselves
and assuage their own guilt...

But to John and me,
the origin of the process hardly matters---
it's only the daily toleration of the clock
that counts for us.

Nothing relieves the fear
and nothing can soothe our worry:
even the elite medical consultants
throw up their knowledgeable hands
and advise us to just stick it out
to the end.

Now that we pass the point of termination
and the life inside starts
to manifest itself on my outside,
it is a time of reckoning
with the uncontrollable process:
I try to forgive a God who has left me alone
and just lets nature do its damage:

I endure the test like Jonah of the Old Testament,
stuck in the belly of a great leviathan.
This time, I am fouled up in the waiting,
plugging my ears from the crushing pressure
of reality.

Week Twenty Four

Believe it or not,
I have always been a person of extremes.

No concept is more offensive to me
than that of mediocrity.
This revulsion to the average
manifested itself in many ways. . .

When I was early on in school years
and learning how to write,
I used my left hand
to form the letters on the page:
this was done to the dismay of the teacher,
who would remove the writing object
and place it in my right hand

Of course, as soon as her back turned,
the pencil resumed its natural spot
in the rebellious left hand. . .

I faced future "rightisms" of school with pride,
as often the lone lefty---
RIGHT-HANDED DESKS
and
RIGHT-HANDED SCISSORS
and
RIGHT-HANDED BOWLING BALLS
on our class trips

All of these things caused me trouble,
but I was pleased to blame it
on my unique left-handedness.

My early left-handed life presented itself
as the psychological stereotype
of the right-brained person:
THE ARTIST
THE MUSICIAN
THE EMOTIVE
THE INSTINCTUAL

I obtained most of these characteristics
from my genetic make-up,
but I learned the rest on my own
(in order to satisfy the requirements that placed me
in the extreme right-brained category)

Whether this was a decision based on pure ego
OR
a natural course of events resulting from chromosomes,
I will never know---

but I ran with the concept
into my teens and early twenties,
where it perpetuated into
an occupational pursuit.

In the elitist realm of graduate school,
I found myself nearly a victim of the average:
there were handfuls of lefties like myself,
all blessed with similar poetic gifts
and in tune with the natural world.

While in pursuit of my English degree,
I desperately donned the mantle
of the complex and verbose writer,
fancying myself a James Joyce
or Ezra Pound

The pages of my papers brimmed with
SYMBOLISM
FIGURATIVE LANGUAGE
ANALOGY
and
HYPERTEXTUAL ALLUSION,
all making for an extremely exhausting read.

In particular, our staid Milton professor
was dismayed by my writing style;
he complained that it was too tiresome
to try to decode, with underlying meanings
exploding over each page
like too many rose bushes
in bloom,
simultaneously

In short, the whole thing really stunk.

So, to get the grade,
I pared down the writing
and took some philosophy courses,
trying to hide my left hand from
the more logical set.

Week Twenty Five

Stuck again in the present, my left-handed self turns
to a new hyperemesis rebound,
with its barely tolerable rounds
of vomiting and fatigue. . .

In desperation, I think,
"Is this whole ordeal a psychosomatic attempt,
albeit a very perverse attempt,
to gain attention as the worst of the worst cases?"

"Hasn't the monster already pared away the ego?"

As I ponder these things,
I start to tune into
a new ailment showing its face:
NOW I feel extremely feverish!

I can't believe that a flu is coming on
in the middle of this mess:
is it a punishment for my thoughts?

By evening, the fever takes precedence
over even the nausea, and I experience a pattern
of sweating and shaking that raises my temperature
to nearly 105 degrees.

I have no more thoughts of self-preservation,
only the primal need to fight whatever infection
takes over at an alarming rate

Our rising anxiety at these symptoms
causes me to the call the doctor, all while
I groan from shattering body aches,
sweating and shivering furiously.

We ride it through the weekend
with doses of over-the-counter drugs,
but the fever swells up enormously
and
then abates
and
swells again

I think we fight the good fight,
but I agree with John to summon my doctor
and get her professional assessment.

The little bird's quick examination seems to
validate my previous thought,
that THE WORST OF THE WORST
is my lot for this pregnancy:
accordingly, the fever spikes, once again,
in the late afternoon...

We rush off to the hospital's high-risk ward
(our familiar hunting ground),
and I collapse into the starchy hospital bed
as the nursing activity around me
begins to surge...

Jenna C. Schmitt

Week Twenty Six

The fever burns a frenzy around me
I have not yet experienced,
even in the earlier weeks;
our little bird watches my vital signs
and the alternately receding
and rising temperature
with anxious eyes.

A theory emerges that my infected gall bladder
gives out under the strain of the
artifical diet and constant vomiting;
our faithful surgeon (in cowboy boots) arrives
and orders another ultrasound of the abdomen
in great haste.

I don't care about the threat of surgery,
I just want relief from this insidious infection;
all I do is turn and writhe all night
in the uncomfortable bed,
I.V. dripping rapidly to replenish
what I have already lost.

The morning finally breaks,
and a surprising conclusion reveals itself:
I have a deadly and yet unidentified staph infection---
it crept into my blood through the PICC line
(the slim blue catheter running directly into my heart).

This has been a terrible threat all along;
it is the risk of an open wound
in such a fractious body:
the only treatment is to rapidly infuse
a very powerful antibiotic,
in order to destroy the tiny microorganisms
already taking residence
in the bloodstream.

The complication of so many factors
leads me to a new level of the word "miserable":
I moan through increased vomiting
and a tremendous burning
in my throat and stomach.

I am plagued by a whirl of nausea, heartburn, fever, and itch---
even the relatively benign issue of skin irritation
(from the sticky dressings on my arms)
becomes a serious matter:
I can't keep my nails away from the bumps,
and burning welts form around the bandages.

Any freedom I felt in the last two weeks,
the feeling of wind and hot light from outside
lifting my hair. . .

ALL OF THAT
is extinguished by the setback,
as I fall back into a vicious state of self-pity,
attempting again to escape
through waking dreams.

Week Twenty Seven

*Hyperemesis is just like one of those visiting relatives
who won't go away---*

*It won't take the hint, even with the initial fall
of pregnancy hormones at twelve weeks;*

AND

It ignores the average statistical stay of twenty weeks;

AND

*It refuses to follow the standard of leaving
by the third trimester
(at the very worst):*

Instead, it brazenly holds on until the bloody end...

*Hyperemesis is just like that acquaintance
you have only by necessity---
maybe he or she is a child of your mother's old friend
or an elementary school chum who keeps calling,
despite your blatant disinterest.*

The nurses, doctors outside the OB/GYN profession,
and casual acquaintances
(such as the grocery checker
who sees my PICC line and wants to know
"What's wrong with you?")
continue to be horrified
at our insistence that this will be
our first and last pregnancy.

They seem to view sterilization
as an extremely sad and drastic mode of birth control,
but WE KNOW it is a vital preservation of
my quality of life.

Adoption is never a good enough alternative to these people,
and they lament,
"How can an adopted child be as much yours
as one you've cultured for nine months?"

We try to chalk up these remarks
to pure ignorance
and their off-hand comments of
"every pregnancy is different"
to a lack of activity in their own lives:

THESE PEOPLE certainly will NOT BE INVITED
to our post-birth tubal ligation party!

Week Twenty Eight

In the outside world,
summer continues to roll by us
and brings all of the seasonal events to fruition:
they are as inevitable as the sun rising and setting
each broiling day in Arizona.

The weekend weddings arrive in succession,
and we attend receptions when I am able:
I suck down watery juices
and the spare appetizer tidbit,
watching celebratory events unfold.

I mechanically extend congrats
to the happy couple, while remaining morose
in my own thoughts.

Usually we sit next to an unsuspecting victim:
this is someone or some couple who is curious,
or just bold enough, to ask us how the pregnancy is going...

My initial reaction is to gloss over our response
and summarize it quickly with the word "fine"---
however, at this point in the journey,
I abandon that polite idea
and describe "hyperemesis hell" in explicit detail

The inevitable reaction is disbelief,
followed by more questions and incredulous looks.
The conversation ends with the start of the buffet line,
when my victims use this moment to escape
the unpleasant thoughts I provoke.

I suppose if I can just spark
LIGHTNING BOLTS
into
fertile brains,
that maybe SOMEDAY my story
will help a sufferer the victims might meet.

I hope they would react
in profound sensitivity toward the afflicted,
and with a heightened sense of empathy
they may not have possessed
without asking me
the initial profound question. . .

Week Twenty Nine

During his weekly check-in phone call,
my father delivers news
that is both sad and thought-provoking.

Just plain old age forces
my ninety-seven-year-old grandmother
into an assisted living environment;
of course, this is for the practical best,
but it is against her considerable will---

Grammy struggles with my aunt and uncle
(my father, being the stepchild, moves aside),
but she finally relinquishes her fight,
due to sheer exhaustion at being
ninety-seven.

I try to imagine Thanksgiving without Grammy,
the Smith family matriarch;
I picture some impersonal catered affair
at a golf club restaurant, with extended relatives
leaving as quickly as possible after dinner.

Each year we gathered at Grammy's house
on Ben Franklin Road, in the cozy town
of Indiana, Pennsylvania. . .

This city is the birthplace of Jimmy Stewart
and a haven for traditionalists, who are
still stubbornly stuck in the 1950s:

Jimmy Stewart landmarks litter the downtown;

WHILE

wooden-floored hardware stores sell penny candy
that is decades old

AND

tinkly little gift shops bear the finest flea market bargains
in the county.

I had such a love-hate affair
with our trips to Grammy's house:
inevitably, I would sneeze and snort the entire time,
due to my nasal allergies and nearly 100 years-worth of
wrapping paper and plastic bags
that she stored meticulously
in the musky basement.

Inevitable, also, were the eccentric joys
of the singing refrigerator and antiquated plumbing---
our favorite trick was to flush the toilet downstairs,
and it would cause the toilet upstairs to shoot water
in the air several feet,
soaking whatever unsuspecting bum
was on the john.

We younger cousins
staged epic plays in Grammy's basement:
during intermission, we listened to 1940s recordings
of the Chipmunks Christmas albums and read
cousin Greg's love letters to his future wife Sue.

In the midst of this family chaos,
our Grammy would sit proudly,
perched on Grandpa's old worn chair
in an equally worn living room.

Family photos and patriotic memorabilia, all from years ago,
peppered the entire rickety house.

As time went on, Grammy heard less
and therefore seldom spoke,
but what she DID say was still precious:
she spun wonderful stories of life in the horse and buggy days,
and spoke of her young nursing career at the schools
and in the county hospital.

We laughed at Grammy's strange attempts
to live in the current century,
like when she unknowingly planted
and then burned
marijuana plants in the backyard,
which cousin Jeff had brought back from Haiti...

She also amazed and scared us with her resilience,
like when we caught her secretly chopping wood
in her early nineties,
as well as driving to church every week
without being able to read the street signs anymore.

Grammy was a solid institution, standing stock still,
while the rest of the world rushed by.

With her passing, I realize that back then
we were too eager to grow up
and too eager to talk
without listening.

And in my current haste
to move on and bear this child,
I am afraid to leave Grammy behind;
I fear that her passage into the next realm
might go unnoticed

It is the passing of an era that will never be experienced again.

Week Thirty

Something strikes me at this point in the pregnancy:
I have gained a sharp comprehension
of the difference between pain and discomfort,
an understanding which
I never anticipated to experience
so early in life.

The PAIN of hyperemesis
is the nausea and projectile vomiting:
what makes it a true "pain"
is that its intensity is beyond my control.

DISCOMFORT, on the other hand,
appears and reappears rapidly
like a light blinking on and off in my brain,
but it is easily circumvented
BY MEMORY
BY EXPERIENCE,
even
BY CONVERSATION

Discomfort is not a focused power, like the penetrating force
of hyperemesis.

Discomfort is my present affliction of itch,
something that many pregnant women experience.
Again, however, mine is a different case
because it results solely from the translucent dressings
that stick to the bad PICC arm.

A penetrating itch rages, and I must scratch it
just to get some pleasure of relief---
but this relief comes at the great price of an open sore
and nasty yeast-like stench.

This event sends me back to the little bird
for the diagnosis of an E Coli skin infection,
which calls for yet another round
of the dreaded IV antibiotic therapy.

To distract myself from scratching,
I remember old discomforts,
like the pressure burns I got on my soft inner knees
from taking riding lessons
in shorts.

I also recall a blistering sunburn I received
when I stubbornly refused to wear any sort
of sun protection in my teenage years---
the most extreme example occurred
at a horse show when I wore
my short-sleeved riding shirt
SANS jacket
in the intense August rays...

I recall that the resulting "farmer's tan" looked quite attractive
with my strapless prom dress.

These memories point to an uneasy balance
that exists between helplessness and willpower:
it shows that I DO have the ability to make any
discomfort worse or better
to a certain degree.

I realize that DISCOMFORT is within
the realm of my control, even when
the PAIN of hyperemesis continues
to runs amuck.

It is this rationalization that comforts me,
as I near the final days
of my first and last pregnancy.

Week Thirty One

As time hastens my methodical progress
to the finish line,
the concept of "baby"
finally rises into second place,
behind our awareness
of HYPEREMESIS GRAVIDARUM.

John and I get to see an amazing 3-D ultrasound
of our little Jay (as we call him), and
I am stunned by the image on the screen
of a real baby, not the ultrasound alien
we are so used to seeing. . .

He has soft fleshy cheeks
and a prominent little snub nose
(a perfect hybrid of John and me):
on camera, we see him make real life,
real time movements, with his hand in a wide-open mouth,
and the other foot grasped in a tightly clenched hand

His eyes flutter open and seal shut right in front of us,
on the darkened computer screen.

This "thing" I have only imagined
finally evolves into OUR CHILD---
left far behind are the days of early shrimp-like stages,

when he actually had a TAIL,
and I swore I could see feelers...

In that animal form, it was so much easier
to resent him for my trouble.

Now as I view him, so solid and so tangible,
I feel some guilt for the early animosity
I had toward my son,
whom I could not immediately view as human.

Now his very real humanity seems to propel us forward,
and we finish the necessary tasks that befit
the arrival of a REAL baby:
John paints the room,
I clear out the guest furniture,
and we finally purchase the
FURNITURE
CLOTHES
WIPES
FORMULA
DIAPERS
that are required.

The flurry of activity reminds us
that quite possibly,
the delayed joy we have hoped for
all along
isn't too far ahead.

Week Thirty Two

I think about little Jay more often
after I see him floating in the warmth
of my own womb:
I wonder if he hears the noise of the storm,
which constantly rages in my belly.

Maybe that's why he pokes and squirms incessantly,
rousing me from sleep and stretching my stomach
into strange conical forms

He jams little active feet up into my ribs,
first on the left side;
then on the right side;
and finally settles back on the left side. . .

Do we have another left-handed extremist on the way?

We call him the "pork chop,"
because his meat is tangible:
all of his throbbing organs are fully formed,
and he continues to grow along with us,
down the same passage of time
that we trudge through every day.

It is now that my dreams become more vivid,
and suddenly they are full of nonsense activity,
like me rushing to feed various species in reptile zoos
or zooming in over San Francisco Bay
in a helicopter piloted by my mother.

The unconscious works "full steam ahead,"
while I furiously process the impending birth
and its accompanying parenthood,
like I'm trying to finish
a last-minute quilt. . .

Jenna C. Schmitt

Week Thirty Three

In the middle of night,
I retreat into our guest bedroom
after being awakened repeatedly
by John's open-mouthed snoring.

I fit my wide body carefully into the narrow bed
and try to settle in for the rest of the night.

But the sheets feel too scratchy and cold
without an extra body of heat and comfort.
Also, I keep trying to free myself
from a strange new positioning
of the IV pole.

Finally, I sleep and dream fitfully
that I am drowning in the clutches
of a steel girded fishing ship,
like the doomed crew
of the Andrea Gail

AND

as the death tomb falls to the bottom,

I JERK AWAKE

With that sudden movement,
I pull the blue PICC line
out of my arm by a good foot.
Used to medical emergencies at this point,
I simply roll over and fall asleep,
forgetting that the artificial food source now flows
into uncharted waters outside of its designated vein.

In the early morning,
we shuffle off to the OB triage unit
(to which I am often admitted
but never leave with baby)
and seek some professional help:

The nurses there are afraid of me---
they won't approach the dangling PICC line
without special back up from the oncology ward,
where the staff is used to dealing
with invasive devices.

I wait and cringe as the line is finally eased out
and then pushed into the vein on my opposite arm---
unfortunately, it goes too far in.

This faulty move causes me to sweat
and experience heart palpitations.

After the chest X-ray returns,
(which shows proof of the line's over-insertion),
the PICC settles into its proper place
and I am once again "hooked up"
to my life source (and the baby's food).

Thus, the perpetuation of the whole darn cycle chugs along. . .

Week Thirty Four

After recurrent irritation
and an ongoing threat of infection,
the PICC comes out of my battered forearm;
the little bird decides it's safer to let me struggle to eat
than to risk the trauma of another line misplacement
or staph infection.

I AM FREE FROM THE IV POLE!

I AM FREE FROM DRESSING CHANGES!

I AM FREE FROM WEEKLY NURSING VISITS!

I AM FREE FROM NIGHTLY "HOOK-UPS" TO
ARTIFICIAL FOOD!

Now, a heaver burden rests squarely on my shoulders:
I must learn to eat again.

Learning to eat sounds like such a ridiculous proposition---
it's an inborn trait and natural urge, right?

That's the theory,
but when that theory has been shot to hell
by the hyperemesis monster,

the practice becomes
EXPERIMENTAL eating.

However, it surprises me
that I don't feel any strong emotion
toward the prospect of food at all,
just a bland indifference
that is strangely troubling.

For me, an extreme "live-r" of life,
food has been a natural extension
of my creative appetite.

I have always swallowed food AND life eagerly,
savoring their wonderful
SPICE
FLAVOR
and
TEXTURE.

Now food is only a means of survival,
and I am just a forced participant in the game of eating.

But I try,
and I see if anything appeals:
eventually, the most realistic approach is to discover
what does not offend. . .

Week Thirty Five

Like Columbus sailing into the New World,
I plunge into the unknown realm of experimental eating:
at first, I recall my old cravings for "forbidden" foods,
largely made up of fat, salt, sugar, and preservatives.

I foolishly decide that this would be an ideal way
for me to assert a new-found control
over the beast...

BOXES of DING-DONGS
HORDES of TWINKIES
BAGS of DORITOS
SATCHELS of FRENCH FRIES
BOXES of NERDS
POUNDS of BURRITOS:

The whole big multicolored mess (not surprisingly)
quickly reappears,
all over our carpeted floor.

The little bird OB expresses her disgust
at my junk food euphoria,
but it is not euphoria at all.

Instead, it is the feeling you get
when you shut your eyes
and prepare to dive into cold water:
I AM JUST TRYING TO GET IT OVER WITH---

I try to fatten up
so that my stomach stops moving so painfully;
sadly, I find that the system can only stand
a few tentative scraps of carbs,
a crust here
AND
a roll there.

Lack of substantial food makes me tired and achy:
more afternoons pass by in the dim cool bedroom,
as I recline with a pounding head
and perpetually churning gut.

Week Thirty Six

MOMENTS OF WAITING FINALLY DRAW TO AN END.

This enables me to forge through a cloud of nausea,
when the heaviness of late pregnancy hangs low,
and the baby kicks and squirms
in its warm prison.

My bones ache and begin to spread,
preparing for the CLOSE reality
of birth.

I still tackle daily errands
armed with the trappings of hyperemesis:
"SPIT" RAGS for uncontained drooling;

PLASTIC BAGS for sudden attacks of vomiting;

BOTTLES OF PILLS to control acid upheaval. . .

Despair lingers on, but it slowly begins to change
into RAW GRIT.

Body Mutiny

Our little faithful bird sets the date,
and she gives us the first goal:
We prepare for a rigorous test,
which will tell us if the baby is ready
to scoot into the real world.

The special day dawns
(perhaps THE DAY of maternal
and paternal reckoning),
and we make our triumphant entrance
into the exclusive cocoon
of labor and delivery.

As always, I heave and vomit this morning,
but the effort now seems noble;
it is a final means to an end,
which will bring both John and me RELIEF.

The test begins and my nerves are steady;
the needle emerges and is expertly placed. . .

My eyes close, but
I imagine its point,
easing down through the
SKIN
FAT
FLESH
MUSCLE
UTERUS
pricking the nerves

and spreading a grimace
across my face.

We await a result for hours;
meanwhile, hope rises up
to the surface of our words
from unspoken thoughts. . .

The little bird kindly calls and relates her "sorry,"
and the trembling turns into tears for me
and silent frustration for John.

But we know to do what is right;
we will put aside discomfort
and we will endure the pain for a few more days,
until the baby can emerge fully mature.

So we inhale and refocus our goal
into the thirty-seventh week.

Week Thirty Seven

In the sweaty depths of another hot Phoenix night,
our phone trills at one-thirty in the morning.

We leap out of our restless sleep, and John grabs the bags
(which have been packed for a month in hope):
we head off to Scottsdale Hospital,
where nurses await our arrival
in OB triage.

I look at the darkened windows of neighboring houses,
as we drive slowly through the winding subdivision,
making our way across Shea Boulevard.

I pity the slumbering people who can't appreciate
the profound hour
which summons us.

It is an appointed and sacred hour,
when necessity demands
the early arrival
of our son.

My nausea rises as I am monitored in the hospital unit:
a humorless nurse, perhaps weary of the dragging night shift,
methodically inserts a cervix-thinning device.

She then leaves us to sleep
and to wonder how the whole process
will unfold.

I snooze only for a few minutes,
but John snores away the hours
with deep, uninterrupted breaths---
biting cramps keep me from true drowsiness
but I welcome them as a sign of tangible progress,
after so many months of empty speculation.

The placid wall clock gradually indicates
the arrival of morning, and I wish for a window
so I could see the break of sparkling sunlight
across the wrinkled mountain range.

I am so close to freedom now, that every labored breath
lightens my spirit.

I have almost forgotten
the thrill of inner happiness
that used to fill my life,
before the storm set in last year;
now I prepare to birth a child,
a thought I had never before considered---

I would have feared this moment just months ago;
I would have analyzed it to death
or tried to deconstruct it to pieces.

Like my old friend T.S. Eliot says,
the end of this journey is one of utter simplicity,
"a condition of complete simplicity
costing not less than everything":
AND
for an astounding second,
I realize that I am sad
to leave my nine-month torment behind
BECAUSE I have experienced a condition of
TRUE LOVE.

I have also learned that
there is no real beginning and no real end
to the curious circular existence
we call life. . .
and that challenges and rewards
often run on top of each other.

Now the birth of something new and wonderful
is so close at hand. . .

Week Thirty Seven, Part Two

At the end of the second full day of induced labor,
the hyperemesis stubbornly holds on,
and it causes me to lose what little lunch
I could choke down, all while I
breathe through contractions...

The little bird checks in
(this time in her scrubs
instead of the brisk white lab coat
she usually dons in the office),
and her demeanor is relaxed
but she is also eager to accelerate
the dragging labor along.

The pitocin comes in, and I am officially kicked into
"active labor" with its arrival;
the result is almost immediate,
with a breath-defying series of
roller coaster cramps
one after the other
in rapid succession
coming on top of
each other and
leaving me
no time
for rest

I wish I could be freed from belly monitors
to pace the hallways---
maybe my steps would fool the uterus
into making a more rapid journey
toward motherhood

BUT

I remain a prisoner of watchful yet detached eyes
at the nursing station.
I know it's just another birth to them,
and that the hyperemesis angle
means little: I am just another bloated
and heaving mother in her ninth month,
preparing to squeeze out a kid.

John and I sense their indifference
and we are thankful for our little bird,
who seems to have taken residence with us
for the remainder of the evening:
she pushes for constant progress checks
and sternly orders an I.V. placement
to ensure hydration.

As the night grows longer,
I am surprised that the rippling cramps
only leave me in a state of discomfort,
not excruciating pain as I had expected.

My worries are very logical---
I might not get any rest
(due to breathing through contractions)
and be too weak to push out my baby next morning.

So the epidural comes in,
and I graduate to the top of the ladder
of priority in labor and delivery:
we are admitted to the maternity unit,
and gladly leave the OB triage well behind us.

THE EPIDURAL PROCESS UNFOLDS...

A brisk anesthesiologist swaggers into the delivery room:
he efficiently arranges the equipment
on a sterile cart, covered with a sterile blue drape;

A sweet-faced volunteer, who is probably
a grandmother to many grandchildren,
dresses the baby's warming station;

The nursing shift changes during these events,
and Patricia, a compassionate
and highly skilled birthing expert,
takes over my case;

THE EPIDURAL BEGINS...

and it feels like jabbing electric pricks down my legs:
it is nastily uncomfortable but not painful enough
to make me gnash my teeth, as I did
during the amniocentesis;
Once in place, I curl carefully on my back,
with limp legs arranged on the bed
(by Patricia since I can't feel them);

I am highly aware of the catheter
in my spine and afraid of dislodging it,
lest I have to go through the whole process again.

THE EPIDURAL CONCLUDES...

With Olympic diving in the background
on our fancy delivery room television, and
I drift into a druggy rest while John arranges himself
on the "dad's sofa" in the corner.

Sometime during the night,
I awake to the screams and groans
of a woman in the room next to mine;
she terrifies me---and makes me sweat
a cold sweat because I have never heard
a human being make such shrill
animal sounds of agony.

I have only heard it in second person,
while watching the Discovery Health Channel.

How will my baby enter the world?

Will I curse the pain of his arrival
like I have cursed my pregnancy?

I pray only
for the safest and swiftest delivery,
and with these inspirational thoughts,
I catch a few more hours of precious rest.

Jenna C. Schmitt

Week Thirty Seven, Part Three

Hazy sunlight streams into my room
after a busy night of medical activity:
this is punctuated by the arrival
of some much needed rain on
this tender morning. . .

Minutes after I am fully awake,
the little bird swoops down and breaks
my water bag with skillful fingers
and a long hook that looks like something
to crotchet with

As she skillfully completes this task,
I am thankful for the fuzzy sensation
and the blockage of any pain---
the faithful epidural remains intact.

But we are disappointed, and I sigh to learn
that once again, my body refuses to cooperate.
The cervix is still stubbornly thick,
hardly a few inches dilated.

Further examination reveals that
the baby's head has come down into the birthing canal;
the poor thing wants to arrive, but he is hampered

Body Mutiny

by my uncooperative surroundings---
the solution is to continue this induction
and toil into the evening hours.

The afternoon brings more storms
both outside and inside our labor and delivery room.

Problems begin to erupt like lava from an angry volcano:
I run a high fever and vomit even more copiously than usual,
and our sweet baby responds by thrashing around
and raising his heartbeat.

The little bird comes to rest in our room,
and her bright eyes dart from my vitals
to the baby's wavering pulse rate;
at first, very little is said, but John and I both
begin to know what she is thinking.

A dreaded infection has set in, and the epidural fails.

I am so, so weary:
FROM FEVER
FROM SHAKING
FROM SWEATING
FROM PAIN
FROM NAUSEA
FROM VOMITING
from being so close to the end of it all:
I feel as if I am dizzy,
riding a wildly spinning carousel,

132

and reaching out precariously
to grab the golden ring---
but it's just out of reach. . .

There is the instant realization,
by all of us involved in this nine-month-long event,
that the baby has to come out NOW!

He will exit by the surgeon's knife
and be plucked out of my abdomen
by several welcoming hands.

Our sparrow has such small hands,
but they are strong, and in them alone
I put my hope, having run out of strength
and the ability to worry anymore.

In haste, we dress for the big event
and I am wheeled into a bright room,
after a rapid trip through twisting hallways.

I scan the walls of this operating room,
trying to remember minute details of the moment:

a red digital clock on the wall marks the time;

masked and smiling eyes look down;

monitors trill and beep for my comfort and safety. . .

There is a painless sawing sensation of knife,
across the place where the baby kicks.

I feel John's hand on my outstretched hand,
which is tied unceremoniously to the table:
I lie in a crucified position, spread out
for the convenience and ease of surgery.

There is cutting and pulling but it does not alarm me
because I know I am at the end
and it is glorious!

AND
IT HAPPENS. . .

A huge vacuum strikes me in the chest
and I GASP---
just like I did in third grade
when I fell off the teeter-totter
and knocked the wind out---HE IS HERE!

HE IS HERE,
and he is a pulsating being
thrust over the top of the drape
which lies across my chest.

HE IS HERE,
and he is red and shiny with flaky dry skin
and so much dark tangled hair
on his round little soiled head.

HE IS HERE,
and I know his profile already from
the ultrasound, with the snub nose
and softly rounded cheeks,
a masterful mix of his father and me.

HE IS HERE,
and I view him with calculated indifference,
seeing only the details, because it is a moment
of incomprehensible disbelief
that he is truly outside of me.

HE IS HERE,
and I am free from the torment of the monster!

This is the thought that brings
tears to my eyes...

Week Thirty Eight

I am a prizefighter beaten to a pulp
by a vicious opponent:
he showed me no grace, even when
I cried out for mercy.

But through the suffering and the punishment,
I prevailed and won the fight.

I think these victorious thoughts
as I stagger to the bathroom
the morning after my surgery,
with a nurse on either side,
each propelling me forward in great pain
to do what is necessary.

This is humility that I have never experienced before,
since I can't even lower my own underwear
to go to the bathroom, and the primal effort of walking
leaves me severely shaken.

Humility couples itself with the realization
that I am hungry and thirsty all at once,
and yet there is no dead weight of nausea
or heavy dread that a round of vomiting is imminent. . .

I have my life back, and it is indeed a wonderful life!

I have a beautiful son and a miraculously loving husband
to accompany me on the next journey around the bend:
this makes me feel giddy, like tripping through a bed of roses,
or dancing throughout the countryside
like Julie Andrews in *The Sound of Music.*

I CAN HARDLY CONTAIN MY JOY!

The sight of my amazing but battered son
does not dim my spirits, even though
I ache to see him quietly fighting for life in the NICU

The struggle to be born has exhausted him,
and little Jay just doesn't get a break;
now he battles infection and struggles to breathe,
hooked to a hideous machine that dwarfs
his tiny yet substantial form.

I blink my eyes, but I can't believe what has happened to me in
a few short hours.

The awful burden of the last nine months
falls away like blinders from my eyes, and the clarity of vision
which I now behold is TREMENDOUS

It's like what people who have died
say about walking toward the light:
peace floods over me, and I laugh and cry all at once

THIS IS THE END AND THE BEGINNING OF A PROFOUND THING.

Week Thirty Nine

It's time to leave the hospital since I've successfully proved
to the doctor on call that I do not have any more fever,
and that the antibiotics have done their job...

A lovely sunny Saturday morning greets us
as I take one final shower in the messy room,
and John gathers our dirty clothes
for the three-minute trek back home.

Our house could be a luxury hotel:
my mother-in-law has worked herself to exhaustion
during our prolonged hospital stay,
and the results before us are incredible---

bathrooms shine and glow with the evidence of very recent
cleaning;

the refrigerator overflows with appealing and fresh food;

floral arrangements grace nearly every room;

and there are even purple violets
next to the oversized bathtub in the master bath...

Everything is new,
and everything evolves so quickly.

I am pleased and refreshed by it all,
but there is a strange level of sorrow
underneath the newness
that is heartbreaking.

Our boy still toils on in the NICU,
wearing someone else's clothes
and being fed by relative strangers:
at home and away from him now,
I have nothing by which to remember him,
because he is no longer inside of me
(as my flattening middle can attest)

The emptiness I feel festers away
at the hole he has left inside.

Why do I feel such a sense of loss?
Am I grieving for much more than the absence of Jay?

The answer is obvious, yet it is puzzling at the same time:
I miss my old sick self that gained such courage
through a battle I had no choice but to fight.

But I know that there's no rest
from the greater struggle ahead,
the quest to accept change
with all the good and bad events it brings about.

The only choice is to reach deep within
and to appeal to whatever source gives us strength,
for the resolve to fare forward. . .

Week Forty

So now we have reached the end,
and I thank YOU, the reader,
for making a perilous journey to hell and back with me.

And since we are at the end,
I guess it's time for the grand sum up,
with some profound thoughts
to conclude this long tale of woe
and triumph.

Hyperemesis Gravidarum was a monster,
an overwhelming force lacking mercy
which continued on to the very end
of my pregnancy:
the unrelenting nausea and vomiting
made me painfully aware of its presence,
every waking hour of every day.

It was never in any way convenient,
and it never was kind:
instead, it put me constantly into a state of unease and misery
that caused my mind
and heart to act out in strange ways...

But it was not a creature without purpose:
it sent me spinning back into memory,
and recollection enabled me to learn
from the past in new and creative ways,
in order to cope with the present.

I have become a true participant in life,
and I am no longer just a spectator:

I NOW HURT MORE ACUTELY
and
I NOW SEE MORE CLEARLY
and
I NOW TRY TO LISTEN MORE CAREFULLY
and
I NOW LOVE MORE FIERCELY
than I ever thought I could. . .

I realize that the awesome simplicity
of true love arises from its origin
within each one of us, and that we are equipped to love
if we so choose,
even from the point of our very birth.

Jenna C. Schmitt

As T.S. Eliot concludes:

"We shall not cease exploration
And the end of all our exploring
Will be to arrive where we started
And know the place for the first time."

Suffering has borne me again
into a fullness of understanding,
which I would have never known
without riding out the storm.

The flame it has lit will burn on
for the rest of my life,
and I only hope that I have passed it on to
YOU...

One Year Later

It's the start of the "monsoon season" in Arizona. Today's late afternoon thunderheads have piled into one magnificent, towering horizon. A massive storm builds steam silently in the darkness, punctuated only by flickers of lightning. Now it begins to move closer to our little part of the desert, and I can hear growls of thunder. This is my favorite time of the day.

Last year, my own "inner monsoon" unfurled: I was pregnant and very sick. But before that event took place, I spent many years prior stuck miserably in a "perfectly sunny day." Mired in the numerous disappointments of life, I surrendered to despair and self-loathing. Then the pregnancy blew in and swept away all damaging preconceptions. In retrospect, one year later, I understand exactly why I needed the arrival of such a momentous storm.

I lost control last year. Control is something I will never truly have over the most profound circumstances. Whether you want to call it a cosmic "master plan," or the Divine, the greatest eruptions in life force us to live outside of selfish desire. After the pregnancy, I learned that I can never take the risk of having any more children. Nine months was all I had of my "reproductive years." There is sadness in this fact, but I am just starting to uncover many marvelous gifts I have since gained.

Today, I am free from old insecurities and live a new life. Now, amazing blessings take place. There are so many unparalleled joys! I delight at my son, a miracle of science and religion, as my husband says. I revel in our steadfast marriage, made radiant by adversity. I marvel at the new and precious friendships we enjoy. I wonder at the advances my case still brings to the medical community.

The miracle of creation continues to inspire me. It's true that my experience with *hyperemesis gravidarum* made the writing of this book possible. So now, what will I do? I will share my story of survival with all women in the midst of their own respective struggles. In particular, I hope to identify with all the miserable morning sickness troopers, as well as those just hanging on, as I did. The story of my book is one of sheer survival. However, in the end, it is truly the gift of "delayed joy" that brings the sweetest reward.